60 is My New 20

The Hayden Diet for the Modern World

Book by Author

Mr. Richard Hayden

Written in March of 2017

About the Book

This book is about my life story of how I live in perfect health. I also tell what I do to look younger to have a young body of a 20-year-old; now that I'm older.

I tell about all the things that I do and how I live my life. I explain what food supplements I take each day.

I tell about what foods I eat and what foods I do not eat and the reason why I don't eat them. I tell people how to fallow my healthy life style and they too will see great results for a healthy young life using the Hayden Diet.

I explain about the major health related problems of today and how it can be turned around. I tell how simple it is to live the Holistic way of life and the many benefits of staying healthy and young for many years to come.

I explain the reason why having balance in life with everything is a major key to having good health and living young. Having the right balance puts us in tune.

I tell about the advancements in Anti-Aging and how a person can look younger and stay that way.

I tell how a high protein diet, with the best supplements, light exercise, the proper sleep and the right amount of play time to take away all the stress; will give people a life of great health and a young body starting today.

Ask Yourself These 10 Questions

Do you need to Lose Weight?

Do you need Hormone Balance?

Do you need a Stress-Free Life?

Do you need a Powerful Sex Life?

Do you need Extreme Energy?

Do you need Great Memory?

Do you need to Live Pain-Free?

Do you need a Life Without Medicines?

Do you need to be in Perfect Health?

Do you need to Look and Feel Young?

This Book Answers Yes to All 10 of These Questions and Tells You How Easy it is to Achieve Them Fast.

∞

Look Thin

Look Fit

Look Young

Amaze People

Live and Be Healthy

Feel Young

Feel Alive Again

And Be Happy

∞

Contents

Continue Next Page>>

Contents Continued

What is Perfect Health?

Perfect health is living the life the way we are meant to live. Perfect health is having cells that keep us young. Perfect health is living life without disease. Perfect Health is the fountain of youth. Perfect health saves us time and money and perfect health allows us to keep up with any generation. Stronger and faster than teenagers.

Perfect health makes us a stronger work force in society. Having perfect health well over the ages of 50-60-80 and even over 100 years old; means we still have a lot of people working, playing and having fun with their lives when their older. This adds a lot of value to society.

Imagine people that are living in perfect health way off in the future. They would be over a 100 years old and they would be competing in the Olympics and they will compete with young people that are only 20 years old. The young one's better pay attention; the older one's have experience. Three life times as much; but with the same health, strength and stamina.

Having perfect health is a chosen lifestyle. Like anything in life; we have to get used to it and after a while things get easier and life gets better. To get perfect health it takes time for our bodies to cooperate and our cells to adapt to improving our health.

Maintaining perfect health also has a lifestyle of its own. These days, it's always keeping up with the newest human testing for Anti-Aging. Researching and Testing Supplemental Health Inventions are always an ongoing research. Doctors and Scientist in their Holistic Fields of study; are always finding ways to allow more and more people to live in perfect health these days, more than ever before. Good health is now affordable.

Some people are old enough to remember how their great grand parents lived. They remember how they lived off basic whole foods to keep them healthy. People back then were not lining up to buy medicine and they were not going to the doctors all the time.

Hard work is what aged them faster and if they had the modern day anti-aging supplements; they too would have lived longer and had perfect health.

Having perfect health these days; you don't hear a lot or even see a lot of people who have it. Most people are far from it. Like with any problem, including health problems; there's always a solution.

People say that an Olympic Athlete is who they think of when I say perfect health. Perfect health is for anyone who puts their mind to it and focuses on having it now. Putting mind over matter will attract perfect health.

The law of attraction is always here giving us the power of thought and the power of healing and to live in perfect wellness for as long as we want to live. Ask and it is given. Ask for perfect health and receive it. Ask for youthful looks and receive it. Think it and attracted it.

Why do most people that are 20 years old; want to live it up, party and have the best fun that they can? Because now is their chance to enjoy their youth while they can.

People have been programed into thinking that by the time they have reached 30 to 40; it's too late. And by 50 to 60 their health is only going to get worse. Sad but true only in their mind. Why? Because I'm living it up right now. I'm still enjoying a youthful life each day.

People like myself that are not conforming to the so called ways of life; are continuing to have an open mind, by always wanting to have perfect health. People who want to live in perfect health; are always searching for the best of the best in nutritional supplements. Now we are doing what the 20-year-olds are doing. Living Young.

People that are in perfect health say that dying young is a thing of the past. People in perfect health say disease is a thing of the past and getting old looking is the thing of the past. No one wants to look older than they are.

As we get older, we still want to look young and we want to have perfect health. Why? Because that's how we live longer and enjoy our lives.

The main part of having perfect health; is living in a lifestyle, that has ongoing maintenance for the body to keep it in perfect health. Day to day maintenance is achieved by normal but good healthy habits. Once these are obtained daily; after a while it becomes so easy that things are done subconsciously.

Like anything, perfect health comes with a price. However; compared to the cost of bad health, the cost is a lot more. Spending $200 a month on good health is a lot better than spending $1,000 a month on bad health. What do you spend on health? Too much!

Just by spending $200 a month on good health; at least people are seeing and feeling the results. The most noticeable results are within 60 to 90 days using all natural supplements. Even with regular use; some people are noticing results within the first week.

The best thing I've noticed over the years, is to set the body up to receive great results. Expect great results and allow the cells in our body to their job, by carrying out the orders we give it and that is to be in perfect health.

Super Humans

There is a growing number of super humans today. These are people that take Anti-Aging and Perfect Health to the extreme.

I'm one of these super humans and part of my journey in life is; changing what Americans eat, one person at a time. Showing and telling people what to do and what not to do; so, they too can be in perfect health and become a super human being.

All Diseases start from the belly, or the gut. This is because there is too much bad Bacteria in the gut. Our gut is our second brain. Our gut brain effects our moods, our actions and our performance. When your gut is healthy; then you are healthy.

These days, when we talk about being healthy; there are many kinds of health to be in.

- There's death bound health
- There's diseased health
- There's bad health
- There's colds, flu's and allergies' health
- There's good health
- There's great health

Then there is the best kind of health to ever be in; it's perfect health. When we are in perfect health; we then are super humans.

This is when there is nothing wrong with you at all; at any given time of your life.

Perfect health is on top of my life's list of priorities. Without it; life is just mediocre, boring and depressing.

When you're in perfect health; life is fun, because your body is youthful and ready for fun all the time.

Taking food supplements for Anti-Aging and to be in perfect health; creates a super human being. When we become a super human beings; there are so many advantages to it.

We have so much energy; we can do just about anything that we want. We become very smart and very fast thinkers. We now have the strength, stamina and energy to be the most creative in our lives.

We now do things that we never thought it was possible. Other people look at us and they are completely amazed at all the things that we can do.

What is a Super Human? An Anti-Ager in Perfect Health.

How I'm in Perfect Health

How I started my journey to living in perfect health. It's been a long road; but a continuous road of good health, that has only continued to get better. Complete wellness has turned into living a young life of perfect health.

I Choose to be in perfect health; there for I am.

I haven't always been in perfect health; when I was a born I had a bad cough, that was very extreme in terms of not being in good health. I was also a fat baby. As I grew up; I had my share of TV Dinners and Junk Food.

Back then we didn't think much about the foods we ate; because we didn't think there was anything wrong.

A lot of growing up was trusting too much on the foods that we ate back then were good for us to eat. There was never any question; as long as we were not dying, it was good to us. However; later on, when enough research had been done; it showed that some American foods that we had been eating, was bad for our bodies.

Most people back then wouldn't see the results until they were 60 to 80 years old. These days, kids are having problems just like if they were an old person eating too much of these wrong foods. Now we have to read the food labels before we eat what's inside the package.

A lot of the wrong foods are dressed up to look really good. Wrong foods can even smell really good too. But don't be fooled; what's in the ingredients? They have all kinds of chemicals and toxins in them. The body doesn't know what to do with them; so it stores them.

Now the body is a storing unit. When chemicals and toxins start to build up in the body; people are now carrying around extra pounds of toxic waste. A walking human dump site. No wonder when some people let a fart; it smells really bad.

A lot of people today need to seriously detox their entire body, to get rid of these toxic chemicals. No one wants to carry around extra pounds of unwanted toxic waste in their body. This is the reason why people are gaining a lot of weight in a short amount of time. People say that they are not eating a lot of food; so why are they gaining more? The toxic dump yard, the gut. People need to take Probiotics and start eating whole food again.

With Organic food; the body normally gets rid of it, so there is no buildup of extra weight. With Organic food; you just have to be creative when it comes to taste.

So now as I was getting older; I ate more whole foods and I found myself on the go a lot.

Back then I was active a lot; so, in many ways that was good training grounds for staying on the move and keeping fit. The more that people sit down too much these days; they get slower, they get fatter, they get dumber, they get old faster and they get lazier.

People that don't move around too much or that sit down a lot; get weaker and their body starts storing more toxic chemicals. Their bodies begin to break down because of the overload. Our bodies may be a miracle; but when it's stressed out; it can only take so much.

However: there is always hope with a strong desire and living the dream to make it come true. If your used to sitting all the time; then bicycle riding is a great way to exercise, lose weight, keep fit, have fun and still enjoy sitting down.

I was fortunate that part of my up raising was to eat whole foods. When I was in the military I was fed a lot of good whole foods. It wasn't until I got out of the military in 1981; that I started to pay close attention to the foods that I was choosing to eat.

I started to only look for good foods to eat; like whole foods and organic foods. Back then the price was more because it was no longer the popular food to eat.

Law of Attraction for Perfect Health

I recall back then there was something stirring from within. Ever since; it's been a driving force and a knowingness. I was beginning to go on the right path to good health and paving the way to my future to be in perfect health for years to come.

Since 1981 I've been very healthy and starting way back then; I didn't even know anything about the Law of Attraction, but I was using it anyway. Back then I would say to myself that; *I love my body and I'm in perfect health and I'm grateful for it.*

With these words, I was using the law of attraction. Now I say it every day. I love it and I'm thankful for it.

I think to be perfect health; there for I am in perfect health. Mind over matter; I focus on being in perfect health and my body has to respond and I am. I think my existence into being in perfect health. I'm using the law of attraction and I'm attracting perfect health to me.

It may seem like I'm repeating myself a lot but; we are what we are thinking of ourselves as and we get what is drawn too us by the law of attraction from our thoughts. So wellness has always been attracted to me from my thoughts of being in perfect health.

Food and Drink for Perfect Health

When it comes to food and drink; there are many things available in the market place. But choosing the best food nutrition is always key to obtaining optimal health. I always monitor what I eat and what I drink.

Over the years there are many foods and drinks I had to give up. Like no soda, no fast food, no GMO food, no frozen food, no soy food, no orange juice, no bread and no chemically processed food. Since the 80s I read the food labels and what I found was that most packaged foods in America are the wrong foods for the body.

Some say I eliminated all the fun in life. What's so fun with foods that make you fat and die young? Nothing; however there still is fun with the type of foods I select.

Here's an example of a snack anytime. Organic grown cored strawberries washed in purified water, added to a bowl with stevia sweetener and raw honey. Mix it up and cover and chill and serve. Another example is my evening dessert. It's all natural peanut butter, raw honey and 70% chocolate bar. I mix some honey with the soft peanut butter; then I spoon some on to a bite size chuck of chocolate and enjoy. I also drink Green Tea, lots of purified cold water and stevia sweetener.

Buy Organic and Eat Less

These days, most people are almost full all the time. This is because people are eating way too much food. When we eat too much food; our stomach is always trying to digest the food.

In the meantime, since the stomach is almost full all the time; the belly sticks out a lot more. Hence the word pot belly.

One main reason people are eating too much these days, is the type of food that they are eating. If it's not Organic food; then the body will not be getting the proper amount of nutrition. Because of it, the body now wants more; because it's not getting enough nutrition.

There are two more reasons why people are eating too much food. One is; people need to take Enzymes before they eat. This breaks down the food faster for digestion and gives the body more nutrition out of the food.

The second reason is; our Cave Men and Women Ancestors. Back then we stored food, or fat in our bodies to survive. This was because we didn't know where our next meal was coming from. So, our bodies became fat storing machines. Today our bodies are still the same.

We still carry on with the same instinct as our ancestors did back in the cave man days. We're not satisfied until we get food. However, we are never satisfied. This is because it's the wrong type of food.

Today there is Black Cumin Seed oil that will trick the body to thinking that it's full and then you won't eat too much and store extra fat. Another is Berberine; it burns fat faster so the body does not store excess fat.

When we eat the right foods, that are high in protein; we only need to eat a small amount. When we eat too much food; then the body works overtime. When the body is always working overtime; the body ages faster.

When we eat less food that is 100% Organic; then our belly will begin to flatten and we will lose weight much faster.

Stop feeding your body a buffet of Toxic Chemicals. Eat only 100% Organic food. Your body will love it and you will be healthier and live longer.

If you can't afford organic food right now; then you can start with buying and consuming more Whole Foods. The fresher, the better. Whole foods mean just that; whole and not in parts with additives.

Eat whole foods like, more fruits and vegetables. When it comes to protein; buy eggs, beans and peanut butter.

These days, you can always start slowly to change your diet over to eating organic foods. A great source of protein is a small package of organic chicken. Some food stores sell this chicken for about $5.00 to $6.00.

The chicken is even boneless, and skinless. This is a good source of protein that will last for about 2 to 3 meals.

You will be surprised how much you will save and how fast you will lose weight; just by not going out to eat, or ordering in.

With just some simple cooking; you can make great organic soups yourself. Food stores sell organic chicken broth and organic chicken. Plus, organic rice and beans and vegetables. Cook them all together and you could have enough food for a week.

Organic foods can still cause Inflammation; so, taking all natural anti-inflammatories will be an ongoing thing every day of our lives.

With all the Medical costs increasing these days; why deal with it anymore. Start eating Organic Food Only.

My Perfect Health and Beyond

Now that my mind and body are in balance; I feel good. I'm well rested, properly nourished and ready for fun. My body knows it, because it's responding to my thoughts and to the proper balance of everything else in my life. But I need more.

Now that I'm in perfect health; I want to look young. I want to take it up to the highest level. Perfect health plus anti-aging at its best to always keep me looking young. The modern day me.

Since 1981; I've been searching the market and testing many supplements for myself to see if they work. When I got my first lap top PC; I researched even more of the best of the best herbs and supplements in the world. It's been an ongoing research of mine ever since.

It wasn't until 2011 that a major shift would take place. Anti-aging breakthroughs that make the body look young. My research was and still is focused on healthy cell research for anti-aging. Repairing the cells; repairs the body. By keeping my cells 100% strong and perfectly healthy; I would have cells in my body that would be the same type of cells found a baby or a young child. Having young cells again would make me young.

Over the years, I have always felt like I'm a lot younger. I always feel like I'm 40 years younger than I am. Not too many people can mentally and physically say that they look and feel 40 years younger. I feel just like a teenager.

The new anti-aging supplements of today in 2017 are awesome. Each of these new herbs and supplements go straight to the problems in the cells and begin repairing and restoring the cells back to being in perfect health.

Since 2011; the costs associated with new anti-aging supplements have come way down. Many people can now pay for the cost to have perfect health by choosing the holistic way and by using all natural supplements.

Over the years I would try many types of herbs. The very first herbs I bought were for energy. I wanted energy before, during and after my gym workouts.

I was then fascinated with herbs and supplements. I learned how to stimulate muscle growth to make me look good. The next thing I took would be herbs and supplements for my immune system.

As time went on I took a lot herbs. I use to take a lot more supplements each day. But now I have narrowed it down to taking the best of the best in a small amount. Some supplements do many things in one supplement.

Having Balance in Life

Maintaining good balance in my life is key to obtaining perfect health. Balance is a big key in my life now. I've noticed in the past; if I was out of balance; then some part of my life or body would suffer from it.

Good balance is knowing when to stop, knowing that I've had enough and knowing the consequences by not being in balance. These days, it still takes a combination of many things to keep my life in balance.

To balance out each of my days; I take the best herbs and supplements in the world and the right amount of each one to consume and when to consume. It takes the best foods and the right amount of foods to consume. It takes the right amount of sleep and when and how much to get it. It takes the best kind of water and how much to consume. It takes the right amount of work and exercise. It takes the right amount of fun and play for my body to enjoy life and be in total balance and feel good.

The most important part of my balance is to continue as I do, saying that I love my body and I'm grateful to be in perfect health each day in my thoughts.

Part of my balance is exercise. I only workout for 15 to 30 minutes. This releases human growth hormones.

It also takes the right amount of sleep. I give myself 6 to 7 hours of sleep each night. Sometimes I take a brief 20-minute power nap to recharge.

When I want to celebrate; I don't drink to get drunk. I limit myself to only a few drinks. Not a whole case of beer or four bottles of wine.

I also limit myself on the computer. I don't want to miss out on sleep or eating or exercising or having fun. Balance is everything in life.

Balance is the key to keeping up and keeping us on the move. Balance puts us in tune with what to do next. Balance is the key to having the right blend in life and making our life most manageable. Balance makes life fun; because everything is in its place.

Having good balance with everything, allows all the cells in my body to be in harmony and in doing so; I'm in perfect health because of it.

Life is truly great when you put balance back in your life.

Another part of keeping balance in my life is to constantly look for things that will make me happy. Having good balance in life and being happy is the key to living a great life of perfect health and many more added benefits that come with it.

When I'm happy; my body responds to my happiness and it allows me to feel good.

The more I feel good; the more I love my body and the more I love my life. Happy cells create a happy mind and a happy body.

The more I'm happy; I know my cells are loving it. Vibrations of happiness resonates throughout my body and manifests within my body to be in total wellness.

I'm directing my thoughts to feel good and to allow my good thoughts to make my cells feel and to be young. The result is a body of a 20-year-old and related to age; that's 40 years older.

Having the proper and good balance in my life has given me the best of health and continues to make me look young every day.

There were times in the past when my body and my life was out of balance. It's like owning a car; but you can't drive it until it has gas. When we get out of balance; parts of our lives are missing. Because of it; things are not happening the way we expect them to be.

Good balance with good expectations brings great manifestations. One of My Law of Attraction Quotes.

Anti-Aging Supplements to Make Me Look Good

With natural supplements, you could say that I've been a human test study of my own. I'm a volunteer. I have been testing supplements for over 30 years and I have never had any bad reactions to any of the supplements.

At the start; some supplements were good and some didn't do anything at all. In order for me to find the best supplements; it took years of researching, buying and testing. Years later I began so slowly narrow it down to a few supplements that are the best of the best.

Early in the year 2,000; I was getting close, but still waiting for scientists to catch up. I was starting to see and feel what it was like to get younger right before my eyes. But I still wasn't getting young fast enough.

Now in 2017; the anti-aging supplements are speeding things up. People are starting to look young quick. Aging is now a thing of the past.

With the advancements in anti-aging research today; people can go from looking like 60 to looking like 20 in 6 months to a year. This is when they have been using advance technology with proven studies that show results. I have pictures of me 10 years ago; I look older and fatter. I think getting younger is great.

I'd say for the last 18 years; I have been continuing to get younger looking. Now I'm more in tuned with my own health. I know my body well and what it needs. All along the way I've been doing all of this without a doctor and without medicine. Just me and my natural food supplements balancing out my life.

When I look back at old pictures; at the time I thought I looked in great health. But only to realize that over the years I was still getting younger looking and healthier. Some of my friends that I haven't seen in years all say the same thing; wow you haven't changed you still look young, what are you doing? I'm Living young.

These days, the pic's I have of me; Sometimes I have to do a double take. I say wow, I really am getting younger. It truly is a dream come true. My life now is so much better. I get to do all of the things I could do when I was younger. It's like going back in a time machine. I get to have fun all over again. Sweet Tears of Joy.

Everything is so much easier to do these days. I'm racing around not even getting tiered out. I even find ways of exerting more energy. I'm on the go a lot. I can get a lot of things done in a short amount of time. Solutions come to me much faster now and the problems just go away. My mind is sharp, clear and quick.

Age has nothing to do with how you look if you look young all the time. Your Forever young.

Sometimes when I come home from a real physical day; I may have a few aches and pains. But within a day or two; they go away. My body renews itself a lot faster. If I get any cuts; my body heals it up very fast like I'm a young person again.

Now that I'm at the age of 60, nothing much has change in all these years. I will still continue to look young and have the body of a 20-year-old.

At the age of 30 people started to say wait till your 60. Well here I am about 30 years later and not much has changed; other than having perfect health.

Now that I'm 60 years old, I'm laughing at all of the Nay Sayers. These are all the people that had bad heath and because of it they had to say something bad to me. They all were thinking that I would end up getting Bad Health. These are the people that never questioned what they put into their body.

These are all of the things that people said that I would end up getting at the age of 60. Now keep in mind; these are all of the things they said that I do not have and will not have, regardless of what they said.

I'm not bald, I'm not fat, I don't have allergies, I don't wear glasses, I don't have poor memory, I don't have high blood presser, I don't have high cholesterol, I don't have ED, I don't have cancer or any diseases.

I don't have an enlarged prostate, I don't have poor hearing, I don't have low testosterone, I don't get upset stomachs, I don't get headaches, I don't get lower back pain, I just don't get all of the things people get that are directly associated with eating the wrong foods. I just don't want to suffer the consequences.

Every year when I have my physical examination testing; my health medical chart always has a listing of all of my systems being in normal rage. In other words; nothing is wrong with me. I'm in perfect health and loving it. The doctor always says what am I doing there? Proving it.

Because I have chosen the holistic way of life; my body loves it. I've chosen the best pure phytoplankton in the world to enjoy living for as long as I want to live.

Taking the best of the best herbs and anti-aging food supplements in the world and eating the best foods, with the proper amount of balance in my life; allows me to be in perfect health and always look young. Life is so much fun when you can always live young.

Detoxing

During my quest for perfect health I picked up a few things on the way. Like when to say no to the wrong foods instead of giving in. Knowing that we are what we eat and know when I have had enough food to eat.

Knowing what the healthies water is to drink and how much to drink. Knowing the body functions the best when we give it the best nutrition. I know now what my body needs and what my body can do without.

Our bodies are like a sponge; we are like storage tanks that accumulate toxins and chemicals.

Every 6 months I detox the chemicals and toxins out of my body. These are stored because the body doesn't know what to do with it. I do a mild detox, because I don't want to be in the restroom all day.

Detoxing the body is a good way for me to know that I'm not storing something in my body that I don't want. Detoxing the body is also good for people who want to see faster results with losing weight. Detoxing is a way to flush it all out.

Hydrogen free water is great way to flush out the body and to make it run most effectively.

Hydrogen Free Water

Hydrogen allows the body to do what it does best; heal itself. If you drink a lot of Hydrogen free water; you now are controlling your bodies destiny. The instant you drink Hydrogen rich water; the Hydrogen is killing free radicals in your body at the cellular level.

People have been looking for healing Medicines; but all along it's been our own bodies that heel themselves. However, with harsh environments and eating the wrong foods; this has polluted the body to where the body cannot fully repair itself.

Hydrogen is one the best natural healers and Anti-Aging Antioxidants in the world. Hydrogen free water is the river of life. Hydrogen free; means that through minerals and proper filtrating, the Hydrogen in the water is now freed up and now the water is rich with Hydrogen.

If it's not Hydrogen free water; then all the other kind of water in the world is dead water. All other kind of water ages you faster and makes you old.

Hydrogen rich water makes cooking taste better. Also, tea, coffee, hot cocoa, smoothies and protein shakes. Now you're giving the body what it needs to be healthy.

Starting My Day, the Healthy Way

How I start my day with the best nutrition and the best supplements in the world. The first thing I do when I wake up in the morning is put all my supplements on the kitchen counter.

The supplements that are in bottles I take 2 times a day. I take my first supplements with my morning shake. I put my second supplements in a small plastic pocket pack that I take later in the day.

The key to having a proper diet is a high protein diet. So, I've chosen to make yellow pea protein shakes for my total protein each day.

To mix my morning shake; I start with my blender and add a small amount of cold purified Hydrogen free water in to it. Then I add Pure Phytoplankton; one dropper full. Then I add 5 seed oil blend; one teaspoon. Then I add Amaranth seed oil; one teaspoon. Then I add ¼ tsp. of Creatine Monohydrate powder. Then I add three teaspoons of stevia sweetener and sometimes, fruit.

Then I add 72 grams of Pea Protein powder and three tablespoons of Cocoa powder and fill the rest up with Hydrogen free water. I blend it up and then I drink it with my morning supplements.

I do not eat soy anymore. It is not healthy for me, so I look for food that does not have soy in it. I do not buy it or consume it.

Most protein shakes on the market today have a large amount of soy mix in the shake. So pea protein is best for me. However, I like to add cocoa powder for flavor.

I take about the same number of supplements that I do for my afternoon supplements and I put them in a pocket pack for later. All the supplements that I take that are in small bottles are in tablet or capsule form.

The next thing that I do is to make two more shakes for the day. One for my lunch and one for the late day.

I make the shakes about the same way. My lunch shake is 72 grams of protein and the late day shake is 60 grams of protein. My shakes are in BPA free containers with screw on caps, that I keep cold.

My total pea protein for each day is 204 grams. I'm right about the level of what my weight is and that's good. A high protein diet is key to having great health.

By drinking 3 shakes a day this showed me how much food we really don't need. We don't need quantity; we need high quality protein as our main food source.

What Are Bad Foods and Good Foods?

Any GMO, genetically modified foods and chemically processed foods are bad foods. Also, foods that have anything artificial in it or have preservatives that contain Sodium Nitrate or Potassium Nitrate.

What happens is the body starts to have cravings for bad food, or the wrong foods and then what happens is the body wants to eat even more of these bad foods and that's all people want to eat.

When a person continues to eat more of these bad foods; the body begins to start storing toxic waste; because the body doesn't know what to do with it.

Well it doesn't take long, because the pounds start adding on and the heavier a person gets. At the same time, many health-related problems start accruing.

People say but it tastes so good. But now you look and feel so bad. This is the price people pay for being so gullible. They just don't know what's good for them. Re-educate the mind to re-educate the body on what to eat; to get the best nutrition out of it.

People give up because they think that there is no way out. I'm living proof that there is a way out. Start eating foods that are good for the body and see the new you.

Stop eating foods that make you fat and give you poor nutrition and start eating whole foods. Foods that are complete and that are not modified or messed with. Whole foods are whole nutrition.

What are good whole foods? All natural, organic, free rage, hormone free, wild caught, home grown, farm fed and no additives, no GMO, no Soy and no preservatives.

A good start is knowing if the seeds are the original seeds. Not modified. Also if the crops are not spayed with any chemicals. The soil gives life giving nutrients for good whole food to grow.

The last thing that makes a good whole food is having a clean watering system for pure growth with the sun.

Organic foods are a lot cheaper than before. Now more and more people are buying the same good foods their family bought for them when they were a child.

Back then it was just regular food; now it's organic food. This is also because more people are getting tuned into what's good for them.

More and more people are growing their own foods. Home grown foods have a great taste and it saves time and money as a bonus.

Is Regular Food Bad?

Most people these days, have no clue to what is going on and why they are not healthy anymore. They are just unaware.

When I go into the food store in America; I pick out what is only good for my body. I do not eat any of the rest of the food that is there for sale. Most of the food in the store is unhealthy; that's why it's so cheap in price. This is one reason why most people buy these foods.

As I walk down the aisles of the store; the first thing I notice is that 99% of the people I see in the store, including the employees, are all over weight. Out of that; most of the people already have some kind of health related problem, illness, or disease.

When I look into the faces of these people and see their suffering; I think to myself that 99.9% of these people have no clue that what they are eating is bad for them. Eating the wrong or bad foods is slowly poisoning these people and causing them to be fat, sick, diseased and die at a young age.

Regular food is not organic food. Regular food is: GMO processed food, fake and full of fillers and additives that are chemicals and toxins that are linked to cancer.

Our bodies are a miracle; but when people keep overloading the body with chemicals and toxins, then the body gives up and starts to break down and die.

When I walk into the store; what I see is people that look like they are zombies. I think to myself; what planet am I on, did they hide all the healthy people.

They look like they are obeying what they think is right. Who are they obeying? The television and the commercials that tell them what food to eat. They are programed to think this food tastes good and it's good for them. Plus, it's now at a low price.

I don't care if it's the cheapest or the best tasting food in the world; it's still poison.

Most people are like the worker ant, or the worker bee; minding its own business and to carry on in society and never to question authority about anything.

When people take food home and prepare a meal; they are combining more of these chemicals and toxins by adding everything together. It's like a chemical and toxin buffet; ready to attack their body.

Stop eating these types of foods and start eating good wholesome foods that are organic and fresh.

Bad Foods Are Poison

Bad foods will slowly poison a person's body. They may not see it or feel it right away. But after a while they will begin to see and feel the symptoms of bad health, just from eating these types of unhealthy foods.

I used to hear that expression a lot when I was young; *oh, just eat it, it's not going to kill you.* It can and it does kill people who keep eating these poisonous foods.

Not a very heartwarming story to think about. But why is it that I see more and more people these days that are sick, taking medicine, over weight and in bad health?

Bad foods are making them sick, because of the chemicals in them. These toxins and chemicals poison the brain as well. So, the brain becomes stupid. People become less smart then they think they are. I know the difference; they make stupid discussions. Since their brain is in a fog; they don't see or know that anything is wrong until they have a major health problem.

There are foods these days that are so toxic; that it's worse than rat poisoning. Some foods are not even nutritious. There made to taste just like food; but there not real. There are some foods that are 100 times worse than then smoking cigarettes .

These days, the standard American family on a Friday or Saturday night will have pizza and soda for dinner. The problem is; most people don't realize that they are only getting a fraction of the nutrition with this kind of meal.

Most of what is in this kind of meal is poison. Chemicals, toxins, fillers, additives, preservatives and all the things that the body does not need.

The standard American lunch will consist of a burger, fries and a soda. If this lunch was all organic; then the nutritional value would be 100% good for the body.

But it's not. That's why it's so cheap to buy. They make it tastes so good and you will buy more and it will make you want to come back for more. What happens is the body now becomes addicted to these unhealthy foods and creates false cravings. People now crave bad foods.

When we see, or hear things like free food, or buy one get one free, or cheap food for sale, or all you can eat food at a low cost; one word that stands out the most is, lies. They are lying to people. It's really poison.

If people really knew what they were eating; they would spit it out, throw it out and stop eating it ever again. Why would anyone want to continue eating poison?

Social Decay from Food

Social decay starts with how you think and what you feed your body.

If you first have the wrong thinking to feed your body the wrong foods; then your body and mind will begin to decay. (Hence, Social Decay)

The American society is in the danger zone of social decay. 80% of Americans keep on feeding their body with toxic chemicals.

They are either unaware of the dangers of what they are doing to their body, or they don't care because they are poor, or they don't know that there is a correct way to feed the body exactly what it needs to be healthy.

This is what happens when people continue to eat bad food: They get fat, their hormones are low, their mind and body are slow. They have poor memory, they are not as smart as they think they are anymore. Their sex life is gone and their happiness is gone.

It gets worse. Their bodies produce more and more inflammation and their bodies store more and more chemicals and toxins from theses bad foods. Now their bodies are all clogged up.

Some people don't like the way they look now; so, they exercise, they go on a diet and they eat good foods again. But they only get very little results.

So, most people give up. They tried every kind of diet, but nothing seems to work; their still fat and sick. This is because they really don't know what's happening to their bodies from the inside.

We all have fat cells and just like our regular cells; they each have receptors, like little antennas.

Normally in our body; our fat cells communicate with the rest of our body to burn fat for energy, growth, repair and general nutrition.

But if our fat cells become clogged up with chemicals and toxins from eating bad foods; then these fat cells can't communicate because the cell receptors, or antennas are clogged up.

The bodies fat cells now are unable to communicate to be burned for energy; so, the body stays fat. We can try all the diets in the world and eat the healthiest foods and exercise until we drop. But if fat cells can't communicate; diet and exercise will not do anything.

Our body does two things; eliminates or stores.

Our bodies naturally store fat to be used later for energy. But when fat cells are clogged; they cannot be burned for energy. So, the body now stores even more fat and people wonder why they don't have energy.

Once the bodies fat cells are unclogged; then the fat cells can now communicate again and the body can now get back to normal fat burning for energy, etc.

These days with modern technology and holistic doctors and scientist; they have narrowed it down to just a few natural supplements to unclog these fat cells.

The most popular one is: Probiotics. Enzymes, Coriander Oil and Berberine all help to unclog and burn fat faster.

Once the gut rot is cleaned out; now the fat cells can communicate and people will no longer be a prisoner to their own body.

Once their body is back to normal and they continue to eat good food; now their bodies are no longer decaying and their minds are smart and fast. Now society is back on its feet again.

You are what you eat; so, eat healthy and live long in perfect health. Social decay no more. Healthy bodies and healthy minds make a strong social society.

Good Foods List

Anything Organic, Farm Fresh and Whole Foods.

Apples, Apricots, Bananas, Blueberries, Kiwi, Mangos and Oranges just to name a few good fruits.

Avocados, Broccoli, Cabbage, Carrots, Cherry Tomatoes, Eggplant, Green Tea, Pea Protein, Romain Leaf, Spinach Leaf, Organic Plain Black or Pinto beans.

Other foods are: Real Organic Cheese, Almond Milk, Organic Peanut Butter, Almond Butter, Organic Eggs and Organic Seeds, Nuts and healthy Snacks.

The best Fish right now is wild caught in the Atlantic Ocean. Best Fish is; Atlantic Mackerel. Most meats should be boiled or broiled. Fried or Barbequed produces cancer causing chemicals.

Good meats are Organic Boneless, skinless Breast of Chicken, or Turkey.

Anything that's sweet should be made with Stevia, or added to it to make it sweet. Candy bars should be 70% Cocoa Bars and Organic Raw Honey always tastes good on, or in most anything.

Note: Anything with Soy in it is bad food and all liquids should be in a BPA Free container.

Maintaining Weight and Calculating Age

At one time I weighed 250 pounds. At that time, I was 50 pounds' overweight. I lost that weight eating whole foods and taking the right supplements. I lost that weight in 3 months.

My entire adult life, my average weight has been 200 pounds. The average weight gain over the years has been 20 pounds on and off. This is a combination of fat and muscle weight.

The nice thing about maintaining my weight over the years; is not having to buy bigger sized clothing. My wardrobe can stay the same and since I know my size; it makes it easy to shop for new clothes.

Another thing that's nice is not having to buy a lot of extra food. The more we weigh the more we eat.

If 60 is my new 20; then when I'm 80; that will be my new 40 and when I'm 105; that will be my new 65 and when I reach 140; that will be my new 100.

Either way I will always be gaining by 40 years younger than my real age. 40 years' younger feels great. I always feel young and ready for life. Every day is a new adventure and another day to have fun. I always have the strength, stamina and energy for anything.

Skin Health

Over the years I have also been paying attention to my skin. I like the outdoors; so I'm in the sun a lot. I use 100% Aloe Gel and 100% Coconut Oil. The aloe allows for fast healing of the skin. Coconut oil is great to use as a natural sun blocker. It doesn't burn the skin; it just brown's it. Coconut oil and aloe gel are best for the skin because they do not contain chemicals.

I go to an indoor tanning place to keep a nice tan in my skin. I've been going to the same tanning place for over 12 years and my skin looks good. People that do not go out in the sun enough; are more likely to have skin problems.

Indoor people need to take high doses of (Vitamin D-3) 2,000 IU a day. D-3 is also a great antioxidant.

I don't use soaps with chemicals in them. I use all natural black soap. I use all natural underarm deodorants with no chemicals in them. All natural mouthwash with no chemicals and I don't use shave cream or gel to shave with. The glide strip on my razor with some water is just fine for shaving.

I shower with filtered water and the best for my skin is Seed Oils and I drink only Hydrogen Rich water.

People's skin is bombarded every day; so, adding more chemicals to the skin is just going to make it look older than it really is. No one likes old looking skin.

Some people say to me; if I'm in a tanning place at least 5 days a week, isn't that bad for my skin? I say no. Most people say I have great looking skin for a 60-year-old.

I also take supplements that help my skin look good from the inside out. I consume organic olive oil; it makes my skin feel soft. I take a 5-seed oil blend of flax seed, sunflower seed, coriander seed, pumpkin seed and sesame seed oils. And the best oil that I take for my skin is amaranth seed oil; which also oxygenates my body.

My body loves these great oils. Some people say are they fattening? I say no. The body needs unsaturated fats from good oils.

By taking all of these oils; my skin loves it. There is a long list of health benefits by taking them. So these seed oils do a lot more than just help my skin.

All of these seed oils are a big part of my fountain of youth and help me to look young. Using oils for my skin makes me feel better and I'm more flexible.

My skin doesn't dry out any more using these oils and my skin stays more hydrated.

What Food Do I Eat as My Day is Ending?

After consuming my breakfast, lunch and late day protein shakes; it's time for solid food. The pea protein is solid; but it's just made into a liquid form.

I don't have cravings; but if I do snack, it's only organic food snacking or some organic whole foods.

I like adding raw honey to natural soft peanut butter and then putting them on some 70% dark chocolate bars. This is usually dessert; but it's also a great snack.

My dinner consists of steamed brown rice, boneless breast of chicken and Broccoli. Also, salad with spinach leaves, tomatoes, avocado, cucumber, olive oil and coconut tree vinegar. Then I top it with white raisins.

Sometimes I'll make some fresh fish or shrimp. It always tastes great with the right organic seasonings.

When fresh fruit is in season; I like eating white or red grapes, cantaloupe, bananas, honeydew, pineapple and my favorite is strawberries, organic of course.

If I go out to eat; I try to stay with the same food groups that I normally eat. If it's pizza; I only eat Organic style. I don't eat sandwiches anymore; most breads are Toxic. Salads are my thing; so, that's what I usually order.

When I'm out to eat; I order iced tea and I do not order any dessert or fries to go with my meal. I pick out from the menu what would be most wholesome for by body.

Usually when I go out to eat; I order less food. I already get enough protein and nutrition from my shakes and supplements throughout the day. Besides. Eating a lot of food only ages the body faster.

I say the healthier the better. My ideal restaurants to go to are; the kind that have salad bars. Why? I already get enough protein from my shakes during the day; so pile on the salad please with vinegar and oil.

Other times when I want a healthy snack; I will eat vegetable straws. They are like vegetable chips with sea salt. I will even eat a whole tomato with some sea salt, or a whole avocado with some sea salt on it.

I don't eat much sugar anymore. I don't want to over indulge myself either. There is a lot of great and healthy foods to eat; but I always stop and look in the mirror and say, I really don't need more.

I try to stop all eating and drinking by 9 pm at night. I especially stop drinking any fluids; I don't want to pee all night. Right before bedtime I take a supplement that grows new cartilage while I sleep. New joints; no pain.

Bicycle Riding

I go out for a bike ride every day. It's great exercise and it keeps me fit. I ride my bike a lot and it has helped me out a lot over the years.

For thirteen years I've been riding bicycles with extreme usage. This is one major part of me being fit and in perfect health. I am pedal power ready to burn.

Biking burns off breakfast, biking burns off lunch, biking burns off dinner, biking burns off the calories.

There is very little presser if any that is put on the body when riding a bicycle. One of the first things people associate bike riding with is; how fun it is. Having fun is associated with riding a bike? Well if riding a bike is fun; then this sure beats seating at home being stressed out.

The second thing that people associate riding a bike with is; it makes people feel young again. Riding a bike to most of us, makes us feel like a kid again and having fun. When we ride around on a bicycle and we are having fun and the stress goes away. Getting your thoughts off the world and allowing fun to come in and fill the void.

When stress goes away; riding a bike is even more fun. It's just you powering you to where you want to go.

When riding a bicycle, the scenery is always changing. It benefits the body and it benefits the brain; because your loving the bike ride.

If you plan new adventures all the time; it stimulates the mind to want to explore something new and you want to go and have fun on a bike. You'll want to ride again.

When we ride a bicycle, we may be moving slower than cars; but we get a chance to see more and absorb more of nature and the outdoors.

Sometimes I like challenges, so when I feel it, I will get up and race down the road on my bike. I have loads of energy. I love racing around town. I even beat cars across the intersection.

These days, bicycles are more popular; but I always use safety first. I still look for bike paths and sidewalks; verses riding in the street. However; the street is fine if it is well paved, clean and enough room for cyclists to ride.

The best 3 exercises for the body are; walking, swimming and bicycling. Bike riding is a big part of me being fit and looking young.

For those of you who run; stop running, your aging yourself a lot faster and putting a lot of stress on the body. Get on a bike and go.

Health Report: Have the Body of a 20-Year-Old Now

These days' people are starting to not like their body too much anymore; because it just doesn't respond how it used to. People wish they had a body of a 20-year-old.

To have a young body again; it all starts with having the proper amount of balance in life. Without balance the body has to work overtime and the body gets tired.

The first thing to get into balance is; to balance the bodies hormones. As the body ages there is a decrease in the amount of hormone production that the body produces. This causes many things to happen to the body.

Low hormone balance decreases energy, increases body fat, decreases sexual desire, decreases stamina and strength, decreases metabolism speed, increases stored chemicals and increases aging faster. Hormone balance is achieved with natural supplements.

Many people look for the fountain of youth because they don't want all the problems of getting old. They want their body to be like when they were young. They want to have the body of a 20-year-old and they want to feel as young as they can when they are older. Now a person can look young, feel young and be young.

The second thing to balance is to know how to balance food intake. To have food balance; the first thing is to choose what food is good for the body. Also avoid bad foods that are not good for the body.

To choose good foods; it starts with a high protein diet; 150 grams to 200 grams of protein a day. No soy. Yellow pea protein is best. No fast food. Whole foods are best. 70% cocoa bar is good in moderation. Also, a note: high fructose corn syrup is 100 times worse than sugar.

The best tea is Green Tea 90% EGCG; good for weight loss. Stevia sweetener is the best all natural sweetener and does not raise glucose levels.

No soda's. Drink Hydrogen free water throughout the day to keep hydrated and to help as a natural solvent to clean out the body. Avoid genetically modified foods and no fast foods, or frozen foods.

Eat only when the body is hungry. If the body is always hungry; then drink more water, than food. If a person is eating out of boredom; then eat healthy snacks.

Buy organic foods to eat and not processed foods. No foods with Sodium Nitrate or Potassium Nitrate. These foods that have preservatives have been linked to causing cancer and or poor health related symptoms. Therefore, eating fresh whole food is best.

The third thing to balance is the right amount of sleep balance. Sleep a minimum of 6 hours, or a maximum of 7 hours a night. Also, if the body is really tired; take a power nap for 20 minutes. When we take a deep sleep power nap; when we wake, we feel like a new person. Most of the time, if your already in great health or in perfect health; you won't need to take a nap.

The forth thing to balance is the proper exercise. Exercise should always be light to moderate and never heavy or strenuous. Exercise should never be more than 30 minutes long. Exercise should be done every other day. The best exercise is swimming, walking and bicycling. The worst exercise is running. It puts too much stress on the body and because of it; the body ages faster. No one wants to look older than they really are.

The last thing to balance is the mind. Mind balance is key to controlling the thoughts that we think. By having good thoughts to think about; then the body will respond to your good thinking.

For example, if a person thinks they are thin; they will be. If they think they're in perfect health; they will be. We get what we think about. When we always think about solutions; then the problems go away.

Best Weight Loss Program Ever

The Hayden Diet; simple and affordable. $44 a month. Knowing what to take from now on will be most beneficial for anyone to lose weight fast. Most foods today are loaded with Chemicals, Toxins, High Fructose Corn Syrup and way too much Sugar.

These foods make you sick and fat. Chemicals and Toxins in the body will cause Cancer and Death. If you still eat these foods and exercise; you will still be fat. Bottom line; stop eating these foods and Only Eat Organic Foods. Now Here's the Hayden Diet.

1) **Curcumin and Berberine:** Anti-Aging, Antioxidant, best for Inflammation and it burns fat fast.
2) **Bromelain Enzymes**: Breaks down food for proper digestion and more nutritional benefits.
3) **16 Stain Probiotics with FOS:** Adds good Bacteria to the gut and kills the bad Bacteria in the gut where Chemicals and Toxins are stored.
4) **Lactobacillus Rhamnosus with FOS:** This one Probiotic is Clinically proven to burn fat fast.
5) **Indole-3-Carbinol with Resveratrol:** Lose weight with Hormone balance. Plus, help protect cells.

I'm living proof that the Hayden diet works. I use it now.

Anti-Aging Diet List for Seniors on a Budget

Anti-Aging and Anti-Stress benefits, Retain Memory, Weight Loss, Pain Free and Live Young Again.

The complete Seniors program is only $40 a month.

1. **Curcumin and Berberine:** Anti-Aging, Weight Loss, Burns Fat Faster, best for Inflammation, Glucose Metabolism and a great Antioxidant.
2. **16 Strain Probiotics with FOS:** Adds good Bacteria to the gut and kills the bad Bacteria where Chemicals and Toxins are stored. Also, great for weight loss and skin cells.
3. **Bromelain Enzymes:** Breaks down food for proper digestion and more absorbable nutrition.
4. **Bacopa Monnera 10:1:** Anti-Aging brain food that is great for Memory and clear and fast thinking. Also, protects Brain Cells.
5. **Ashwagandha Extract:** Anti-Aging, Anti-Stress and Overall Good Health.
6. **Collagen Hydrolysate:** Rebuilds new Joint Cartilage. Younger skin, thicker and healthier hair, stronger nails and no more pain.

Bonus: Spray Magnesium on skin for proper dosage.

Authors Closing Thoughts

These days, because of the toxic build up inside people's bodies; this is causing even more problems when they want to lose weight and balance out their hormones. However; once the body is detoxed, then the weight loss is obtained much easier and hormone balance is then returned.

The toxic that builds up inside people's bodies are from the chemicals that are in the wrong foods, or bad foods. Some people say well a small number of chemicals in the food is not going to kill you. They are dead wrong. When you add up how many chemicals are in each food and then you put them all together to make a meal; now you have a lot of chemicals that can be harmful to the body. If you are eating these types of foods every day; then you are at an even greater risk of health problems.

As people age, there are certain things that the body has less of. Less sex drive, less energy, less memory, less strength, less stamina, less muscle, less hormones, less oxygen and less peace of mind.

Some elderly people say; we work our entire life to have less of a body and less of a life to enjoy. Who designed this body? Now we can reverse all of this by having a great body to live in for a long time and in great health.

It may sound like a magic potion, but once you start reversing everything back too normal; you are now like a new person. You just added 40 years to your life. However; your back better than normal. You are super human with complete sex drive and total energy. You remember everything, you have the strength and stamina of a young person and the muscles to keep up. And you now have the correct hormone balance and an oxygen rich body to live a young life again.

Over the years, the people that I've talked to about my life and all the things that I do to stay fit and in perfect health; say well good for you, or your just lucky. But now that I'm getting a lot older and I'm having even better results; people are starting to listen to me and want to know what I do and how to live in a life of perfect health and how to have a young body for as long as we want.

People see the results I have and they want the same results for their body too. So now people are calling what I do; *The Hayden Diet, for the Modern World.* Take what I take and live longer, younger and healthier.

I've done all the research, I've been the human test subject and the results are, I now have a life of perfect health and I have a young body because of it. I have all the proof and now people want to see their own proof.

You're never too old to live young and be in perfect health. See for yourself and start today by living a new life of being young again.

There are so many benefits every day to having a body of a 20-year-old. I don't get tired unless I need some sleep. I can do many things in a day and come home and I'm still not tired. I keep on the move a lot more then when I was young. People are amazed on how fast I can get things done with childlike energy that keeps going.

Because I'm active a lot, I stay in fit. However; I tell people to exercise every other day; because some people's bodies will not be able to exercise every day. Besides; exercising every other day, is only 3 and a half days of exercise a week.

Now for me; I exercise every day, because I ride my bike every day and I work out a different body part each day with weights. Some days I will work out my upper body and some days I will work out my lower body.

My energy has increased to where I say wow, I never knew I could ever have this much energy. My sex life is like being 20 again, but way more intense and powerful. The desire for it is awesome. The drive is long, rock hard and the stamina is great. No ED for me.

In closing; in the future, the health advancements will be so far ahead that we will know what the body needs and how to repair it with the greatest of ease.

My last and ongoing research is for anti-aging. I will be continuing my research on how to keep healthy cells in our body so we can live as young as we want.

I love my life and I love my body. I know that you will love your life and your body too; once you start seeing and feeling the results by living in a new lifestyle of using the Hayden Diet and eating only Organic foods.

When people's lives are in balance; they live happier lives. Give the body what it needs to repair itself to be young again and live as young as you want.

It feels good telling people about my life and it makes me happy knowing that I'm sharing my real life story of great health to the world.

I'm not telling people that the Hayden Diet works for all people; but it works for majority of people who want the best health and to live young. The More You Feed Your Body Antioxidants; The Longer You Live.

Always Love to a Long and Happy Life of Perfect Health. *From Author Mr. Richard Hayden.*

60 is
My New 20

The Hayden Diet for the Modern World

Book by Author

Mr. Richard Hayden

P.O. Box 257
Palm Springs, Ca. 92263

To Get a $15 One Year Membership

For Monthly Holistic Health News Updates

To Your Email Address; Go to:

PerfectHealthAlways@gmail.com

Notes: